The Thoughtful Diet

Lara Buchanan

I would like to dedicate this book to the two people who, more than anyone, are responsible for all my thoughts
.....

Mum and Dad

Before the book …

For years I knew there was a book inside me, just waiting to get out, and I hoped one day I'd be able to say … "I've written a book" … me !

I never, ever, thought of selling a book. I always saw my mum and dad, close family and friends, just borrowing the only copy … mine.

The book would be passed around and they'd like it because it was mine, and they'd be happy to share in my achievement, even though probably biased.

The fact that other people could perhaps read the book made me realise I had to think about everything differently.

I do believe that in order to write a book you have to enjoy reading, and I'm not a reader … so I'd encountered my first hurdle.

I find it hard to remember storylines while reading, and my imagination simply switches off, so I have to keep flicking the pages backwards and forwards.

If that's not enough, I had absolutely no idea what I was going to write about.

Let me be honest … in terms of filling a book I wasn't sure I knew enough about anything.

There had to be something that I felt confident and passionate about, and there is ...

Losing Weight!

Now on that subject I'm all knowing, a master, and an expert. I've lost so much weight over the years I should be invisible ... ha ha!

The trouble with losing weight is that somehow we just keep finding it again!

I digress, so coming back to the book ...

I'm told I'm a good verbal storyteller, so I thought maybe if I wrote my book in a similar way, then there'd be a chance that readers might enjoy my thoughts.

Two things I still had to do ... decide on a title, and go back to 'Fat Land'.

At last my little book has evolved enough for me to be happy with its content.

I've been on a long journey to get to where I am.

Welcome to my world of ... **_The Thoughtful Diet_**

Thoughts on ...

- Reasons for

- Beyond acceptance

- Further reflection

- Carry your own weight

- Past desperations

- Present day solutions

- Future expectations

- Your past lies just ahead

- A forever kind of diet

Reasons for …

As you travel through this book my thoughts may, or may not, start to make sense. Either way, please have a stroll … there's no hurry, and no pressure.

So ... why would I want to impose yet another book about all of this stuff onto those of you who probably know it all anyway? These books do all kind of say the same thing don't they?

Even though they may be factual and well written, there is a lot of repetition and same old same old … yawn, yawn.

I also find it can all get a bit "Oh no, not another Diet & Fitness DVD on the TV'" (especially just after Christmas), reminding me once again that I'm overweight.

You may well ask … have people got nothing better to do than go on and on about obesity, and why are those same people normally slim?

It did not make any sense to me that if we have all the information about what we need to do, then why are we not using it, and why are we still overweight?

For the past 18 months my head has been full of thoughts on what I could eventually write about in a positive way. It was like having a 500,000 piece jigsaw, all in tiny parts, with no sense of order at all, and the last piece being missing altogether.

I suddenly realised the last piece I needed before I could write my book, was that I had to put on weight again!

This time though, it was my choice … weird!

In all my life I have never heard anyone say that they choose to be fat. It just creeps up on them … me included. We go to bed one night and wake up four stone heavier, at least that's what it feels like doesn't it?

The experiences and stories I'm using in this book are mainly about weight loss, (because that's what I know about), but the comments and observations in '*The Thoughtful Diet*', might also help in other situations.

It is about accepting yourself, or your weight, as it is now, (if you're happy of course), and offering another perspective if you're not.

Whether you are fat or thin, young or old, male or female, fit or unfit etc., etc., 'The Thoughtful Diet' could be relevant for you.

Hopefully something you read will flick the switch that allows you to take back control.

We all have our cards dealt to us, and they belong to us and us alone … no one walks in our shoes.

I've spent many hours trying to think of a scenario where there was someone out there who had been granted a get out clause, (apart from a serious medical condition). So far I have not found you, but if you are out there then I would like to say I'm sorry.

You are unique, and my wee brain never thought of you.

Beyond acceptance ...

We have a major crisis in the UK, that's now at the epidemic stage, and it's called 'Obesity'

It's not comfortable reading or writing about it, yet I think it's important, and should continue to be highlighted.

Recent media attention is raising awareness of it, and should help in the realisation of where we have come from, and where we are headed if we don't make some changes.

This book is about encouraging you to change how you think, so let's get the heavy stuff over with first.

It doesn't seem that long ago, where if you were a 16+ dress size you had to go to an outsize shop, and it wasn't somewhere younger people went, because it was the older generation who had 'plumped up', so to speak. The majority of kids were not overweight, and besides that, going to an outsize shop wasn't cool!

The clothes were larger so they obviously used more material, and therefore they were more expensive

Makes sense doesn't it?

Here's a wee story ...

While shopping with my mum I fell in love with a sweater. From a distance I knew it was meant for me, and I approached very quickly to have a better look.

It was even more gorgeous up close … white crochet, long length, and buttons going all down the back. I had to have it, it was love at first sight. I picked out a size 12 (for when I'd be back in Slim-World), then checked out the price … £22, and worth every penny.

Then I spotted that it was available from size 8 to 22, yet the price was just the same. How could that be? One size is seven sizes larger than the other, obviously using up more wool, so how come it's one price for all?

Why should someone who's a size 8 pay the same as a size 22? I don't get it, it doesn't seem fair.

I've been a size 22, and worked really hard to get to a size 12, yet in monitory terms nothing changed.

If someone is living their life overweight, then what incentive is there to lose some pounds when all around them everything is geared up to accepting obesity. We are being encouraging and accommodating.

We do not wish to hurt people's feelings, and we are afraid to be honest, which to me just doesn't sit right.

This way of thinking is currently creating so much sadness further down the road.

For example, the demand for outsize coffins is on the increase. The same applies for extra-large burial plots, and I was recently shocked to hear that as far as cremations go, there are instances of limbs being removed so that the body and coffin can fit into the furnace.

I hope we never see an outsize funeral parlour appearing on the high street, and yet the warning signs are there, but being ignored.

It's even more heart breaking that these instances are not happening to an older age group. They are younger people. Sons or daughters of parents who have lost a loved one, and could now be hit with the double burden of a heavy emotional loss, and possibly a much higher financial cost.

Do I accept that everyone has the right to choose to stay overweight … absolutely!

Do I think it right that it seems to be encouraged … definitely not!

Some people are born really tall, others really short. They have to buy in specialist shops to get clothes that fit, and yet it's not even their choice … that's how they came into the world.

If we choose to stay fat, or live with obesity in our personal lives, and want to continue shopping for extra-large clothes, then maybe it's right that we should pay more!

Outsize in life means outsize in death.

Children should not be obese.

As adults and parents we are providing the food, which therefore makes us the feeders, and that is surely beyond acceptance.

Further reflection …

This section is all about looking at things from a different angle, (which might help to change your thinking), so I would like to tell you another story, and for me it's probably the most poignant. I urge you to real y think about this one.

One of my dearest and best friends, now gone, who I always described as 'a gay Billy Connolly', once asked me this question …

"You know those anorexic folk, and how they get sent to councillors and psychiatrists? Why do they no just get sent to an opticians? How do they no see that?"

It took a few seconds for what he had just said to sink in. I could not believe he had asked me that, and yet, I found I agreed with his thinking!

It's not just people who are severely underweight that don't see their true reflection, it's the same for those of us who are overweight as well!

We fail to see the trickle of pounds going on, or coming off. It's such a slow process that our reflection in the mirror never seems to change, but it's a bit like wrinkles … suddenly they seem to just appear overnight.

If you have ever watched programmes about excessive hoarders, then you'll know that you see people having to climb over 'stuff" just to get to another room.

How do they not see all that clutter?

More importantly, how do their family and friends not notice, or at least be honest with them, about all the things piling up.

Obesity has similar traits.

You don't see the weight piling on, and your close family and friends either don't notice, or simply choose to say nothing, as they don't want to hurt your feelings.

Anybody you have not seen for a while will notice your weight, and they are likely to tell someone else about how much weight you've put on since they last saw you. However, they'll still tend to say nothing about it directly to you.

They will tell you if you have lost weight, but lose too much and once again they won't say how thin you are.

If we, and those closest to us, don't notice, or choose to ignore the trickle of extra weight, and other people who do notice still say nothing, then what chance do we have for realization?

This journey is a reflection of yourself … begin to see a new one!

Anyone who has ever dieted can tell their story about what made them decide to lose weight.

It may be *that* holiday or wedding photo', or perhaps a video recording of a family event, that makes them take notice.

They are shocked because they hardly recognise themselves.

I remember seeing one of my holiday photo's, which in itself was a rarity, because I shied away from the camera when I was really overweight. Honestly, I had no neck, and I looked like a tortoise who'd drawn its head into its shell.

There I was, me looking back at me, and four stone heavier!

When my husband saw the picture he said to me, "If I'd realised you were as fat as that, I would have said something". I replied that, "If I'd known I was as fat as that, you wouldn't have had to!"

We, as the weight carriers, have no excuse. We are the ones putting the food in our bellies, and we are the ones having to go up the clothes sizing ladder. We cannot plead ignorance.

My dad was the only person who continuously reminded me that I was growing larger. He'd tell me it was about time I got some weight off. My dad passed away a few years ago on Easter Sunday. I miss his laughter, and his honesty. He never stopped looking at his daughter's weight, and always took the time to comment.

I guess that's what 'The Thoughtful Diet' is all about … facing the truth, and deciding it's time to make some changes. I'd like this book to be a huge mirror that allows your true reflection to always look back at you, and act as a trigger for change.

Are you ready to de-clutter yet?

Then the next bit, *'Carry Your Own Weight'* might help.

Carry your own weight …

When we booked our summer holidays I was 13st 13½lbs, and my clothes labels read size 18-20.

I was well rounded, literally.

At last, almost ten months later, departure day arrived, and I was so excited because I now weighed a healthy 9st 12lbs, and my clothes had shrunk to a size 10 jeans, and a size 12 above the waist … wow!

My husband did the usual check on the baggage allowance. He stood on the bathroom scales by himself and got his own weight. Then he picked up my suitcase to see the difference, and said "your case is 2kg over the 20kg limit"

What?

I thought, how can it be that I had lost loads of personal weight, (27kg in all, and more than my total baggage allowance), and yet I had to remove two pairs of shoes I really wanted to take on holiday!

It got me thinking. If airlines assume an average weight per person, and we're all getting heavier, does that mean they will have to decrease baggage allowances?

Not only that, but as we become fatter, and our clothes get bigger and heavier, we'll have even less clothes to try and fit into our allowed suitcase!

Now I don't know about you, but I struggle to get down to my 20kg bag allowance already. We girls enjoy the dressing up part on holidays, so please … this can't happen!

The solution is for everyone to get lighter! And who knows, this might lead to an increased allowance, and then … we could take more holiday shoes!!!!

Carrying our own excess baggage weight is not comfortable. Yet, as it goes on pound by pound we get used to it, and yes, sometimes we even forget it's there.

You only have to think about carrying your weekly shopping. You do feel the extra weight.

Our bodies have the ability to evenly distribute weight, so sometimes it piles on and we are unaware of it, or we choose to ignore it.

A lot of health issues can be directly linked to being overweight or underweight, so we have to find the middle ground.

My mum, who is 82 and does no exercise, well apart from the remote control, (sorry mum), and a weekly outing to do the supermarket shop … lost 16 pounds in about four months!

Mum had struggled for a while with a sore leg, and no real idea of the cause, yet the fact she took off some weight made her more comfortable.

Her leg didn't have to lug the extra 16lb weight around with every step she took!

I remember having to walk up a hill to get back to my car, and by the time I got there I felt that breathing apparatus should have been on hand.

A few months later, after losing some weight, the car was parked in the same place, and when I actually stood beside it, having yet again climbed the hill, I realised that this time I was not out of breath!

To be honest it was really just a steepish slope, but when I'd been carrying the extra baggage it had felt like a hill walk.

When you start to manage your weight, you achieve more than just looking better. You will be amazed at how other things will improve, because no one else carries your weight … only you.

Your shopping bags are yours … no one else's.

You have to take ownership!

You don't have to try to put on weight … it takes no thought, it will just happen if you let it.

The only people I know who choose to put on weight are actors and actresses, and of course Sumo Wrestlers. They may need to put on a few pounds for their role, but you'll notice they always choose to lose it again when filming finishes or their career ends.

That part takes thought and control.

You weigh right now exactly what you want to weigh. Do you want to change what it says on the scales?

Past desperations ...

Once we decide to take on board that changes are necessary, then desperation can take over, but that can work in our favour and spur us on.

It can also cause us to simply flap about and do nothing but panic.

We always go back to the past. We remember all the other times when we've tried to lose weight and failed.

When I realised (after looking at that photograph) how fat I'd become, I was desperate to do something.

Twenty years had come and gone, and yet all of the fat had stayed with me ... unasked for I may add.

I went to sleep one night, and woke up fat.

My book title at that time would have been 'How to gain 4st & become 5 dress sizes larger without even trying!'

Realisation slaps us in the face, and suddenly, as if by magic, we get it, and can do whatever it takes to fix it.

 We suddenly have an awareness of our self and we run with it ... at least for a while anyway.

I've had a few slaps in the face regarding my weight ... maybe I just enjoyed being slapped ... ha, ha!

We seem to have this ability to forget feelings such as desperation.

They apparently just disappear, and yet they are lurking in the background, waiting for the next reminder … a memory, a photo, a reflection.

Embrace desperation, it can be a great motivator, but needs to be kept in its proper place by clarity of thinking.

Relax, and chill out … the good stuff awaits!

Present day solutions ...

Take a moment to smile ... the best is yet to come!

If ever there was a time that's giving us everything and more to achieve success, it's now, but we have to think about the 'How' part.

Everyone who has achieved their goal of dropping a couple of dress sizes has something in common... they did what they had to do with the correct tools.

Here are some helpful pointers. I hope this list is well used.

- Clarity of Thinking

- The Why

- Choosing the How

Clarity of Thinking:

By now hopefully you have read, (and maybe have an understanding of), some of my thoughts, and have decided that your time has come.

You have taken ownership of your current situation, and decided you've had enough ... it's time for change.

If you're really not in that place yet, then slow down, and think some more.

All my ideas are linked, and step one, Clarity of Thinking, is the one that will bring all the others within reach.

This is all about your timing, so no pressure … read on, and when you're actually ready, my thoughts will always be here ….waiting. They'll never go away.

All you have to do is change some of the habits that lead you to your addiction to Fat Food.

I feel another story coming on, that's not like me ... ha, ha!

My mother-in-law did not like chocolate.

I repeat, my mother-in-law did not like chocolate ... we didn't even buy her any at Christmas time!

However, after being diagnosed with cancer she was in hospital for a while.

One night, while we were visiting, she said she just fancied some chocolate, so my husband went to the hospital shop and bought her a small bar.

This led to us taking in chocolate at every visit, (which at the time was nightly), and boy did she enjoy!

When she got out of hospital this is the story she told us.

While sitting reading one night, she realised that it was 5.55pm, and the local shop just across the road closed at 6.00pm. She had no chocolate! She jumped up, put on her coat and shoes, and got half way across the road when she thought … "What am I doing, I don't even like chocolate", and she went back home to a cup of tea.

The chocolate habit had, and still was, trying to take away her control.

The Why:

This part is all about why you'd rather be slimmer etc., why you'd love to drop two dress sizes … you get my drift?

The journey you're going on will take some time, and it largely depends on where you are on the road today.

Imagine if you were to win a holiday that allowed you the choice of Blackpool or the Bahamas. Which one would you choose?

The travel time to the Bahamas is obviously longer, with more chance of delays and things not going to plan. You do everything you can to prepare, and you make allowances to make sure you get that flight.

If suddenly there's an announcement of a two hour delay do you say "that's it" and go home (via Blackpool)?

Or does the thought of the Bahamas mean more than a little bit of inconvenience, and you decide it's worth the wait?

That's how you need to view your weight loss journey.

The heavier you are, the longer it will take.

You have to keep thinking about the destination, and why you chose to go there.

All the other stuff is so much easier when Clarity of Thinking, and The Why, are used together.

The How:

There are so many options out there that it can get a bit confusing trying to decide which method to use to help you lose weight, so let me simplify some things.

To lose weight you have to consume fewer calories. Every weight loss diet is formed on that basis.

I repeat every weight loss diet is formed on that basis.

It is a personal choice which one suits you best.

There is a great book available which I have used called 'The A - Z of Calories'. With just this book I took off 42lb in weight.

Some good news … a calorie is a calorie is a calorie.

50 calories of chips is the same as 50 calories of lettuce leaves … it's simply the volume of food that changes.

There are no 'Fat Foods', just foods with more, or less, fat content. It's us that turns the food into body fat by having far too much of them.

When I was counting calories and I had to make choices, this tip helped me! …

Imagine a buffet table in front of you with all your favourite foods. It looks great, and no food is forbidden, you just have to choose.

There is only one condition … you have to keep within your recommended daily allowance.

Any programme will tell you what your allowance should be in order for you to lose weight.

You have to decide what you would like to include.

For example, if you are allocated 2000 calories a day, and one Mars Bar is around 260 calories, then you could have 7 a day and you'd probably still lose weight. But remember, you can't eat anything else as that's your allowance used up.

I am in no way recommending that your diet should consist only of Mars Bars, that wouldn't be all that healthy, and you'd probably be put off chocolate for life! I just want to let you know that within the foods you love there are no taboos. It's eating excess that makes you fat.

There's room on your buffet table for a bit of everything.

It's up to you to choose your calories wisely, and being in control of your food lets you enjoy eating it even more.

All you need is a calorie book, your bathroom scales, and your own self-motivation (your Clarity of Thinking and your Why)

All diets work if you work the diets.

On one of my other weight loss journeys I chose Weight Watchers, and got rid of 56lbs in weight. I enjoyed the classes and did everything I was told to do.

This suited me, as I enjoyed the banter, and found it helped by being around people who were thinking like me.

While with Weight Watchers I bumped into someone I hadn't seen at the classes for ages, and she was still fat.

Her excuse for giving up was the cost of classes, which at the time was £4.95 per week. I suggested that was nonsense, and that it cost more than that per week to put weight on! No one can really say that going on a healthier eating plan will cost a lot more financially, it's just not true.

Trust me, I know. A lot more is spent on the stuff you are eating right now, (crisps, chocolate, cakes etc.), and when you do slim down, you will have extra money to go towards your new wardrobe!

Other slimming clubs work as well, and in general all of them teach you the right way to maintain weight loss.

Fast diets are only recommended, and only work, for those lucky enough to just need a few pounds off.

The best way is the slow, consistently planned, long term way of a 1lb or 2 per week. It all adds up, and the results are more likely to stay with you for longer.

Yet another bit of good news! ...

I believe it's easier to take weight off than to put it on!

It took me years to put on 4st, and yet it only took me about 10 months to get rid of it. I rest my case. Again, all diets work if you work the diets.

Whichever one you choose, my advice is that, for at least the first couple of weeks, you do everything correctly. You will be amazed at the results, and the scales will prove its working.

Do what the successful people recommend, and you will be successful.

Going hand in hand with eating less calories is the bit about doing more exercise. I prefer to use the words "move more", because when I was at my fattest, even the word 'exercise' made me sweat, and I was far too embarrassed to go to public places like gyms.

Think about what you're eating, lose some weight, and simply move more than you do just now.

If you are taking laundry upstairs, then make two trips. If you're making coffee, then walk from your couch to the kitchen twice.

If all you do is double the little bits you do just now, then that in itself will be of great benefit to you, and you won't even really be aware of any great extra effort.

Clarity of Thinking, The Why, and The How, together will give you the formula you need, to get you to where you want to go.

Eat less & Move more … easy peasy! That's all you'll ever have to do!

Future expectations …

When we decide to actually do something about our weight, then pressure comes hand in hand with that decision.

We do not want to fail, so we start out with great intentions, and then for some reason we hit a brick wall.

Our extra weight has been carried around by us for such a long time, yet suddenly we want to get rid of it all so fast that our patience seems to disappear.

We can go for years and never stand on the dreaded scales, but as soon as we 'diet', they become the main reason for our failure!

Why you decide to do something about your weight is more important than the How you lose it, but they need to work together in the formula.

Everyone starts with the 'Feel Good' factor, and is proud of themselves when they start. It's the keeping going that's been hard till now.

It's what you are emotionally about, and what goes on in your head that holds you back.

The good news is that you can change!

This book has, I hope, already got you thinking a bit differently, and your expectations may be much easier to aim for.

Once you accept that changes are necessary to achieve what you want, then the path ahead is easier, but hold on tight it can get bumpy.

You should have truly de-cluttered all the stuff that was holding you back.

It's now time for forward thinking,

Be proud of your achievements.

Even the fact that you've chosen to read 'The Thoughtful Diet' proves that you're looking for a new way to change how you look and how you feel

Be realistic, there is no rush, you choose your destination, and the length of your journey.

I promise you that if you keep looking ahead, and thinking about what it's going to be like when eventually you get there, then it will be a much smoother trip.

Use your imagination, and buy the dress that's two sizes smaller.

Put it on display in your bedroom … it worked for me!

Remember your thoughts when you woke up one morning and decided you wanted to be slimmer?

You wanted to drop a couple of dress sizes.

Has that decision changed? … It hasn't, has it?

If you're overweight and were to ask yourself the same question every morning:

Would I rather be slimmer today?

The answer would always be ... Yes!

Or ...

Am I happy going to sleep fatter than I was yesterday?

The answer would always be ... No!

All that happens is that sometimes we revert back to the old thoughts, the ones that kept us overweight in the past.

Once you re-visit your thinking, you will simply start to move forward again, taking all the good stuff with you.

Your expectations are back in place, so continue to keep your reasons for Why directly ahead of you.

Remember, the Bahamas never change their location, it is your thinking that moves, and sometimes you just forget about how much you wanted to go!

Your past lies just ahead...

April 2013, the time has come …

We've travelled through most of 'The Thoughtful Diet',
and now we must go into the last phase …'Your past lies
just ahead'.

That statement in itself was a close contender for my
book title.

By now you know that you've choices to make, and at
this moment in time, if you are ready to do so, then I
hope my book helps give you a little helping hand.

If you've taken the time to think about your weight, and
you've had a good de-clutter of your fat thoughts, then
you should now be able to move ahead.

Today is now, and the fact you've stayed with the pages
of 'The Thoughtful Diet' means you have done well
today. Give yourself a round of applause … ta dah!

With your clarity of thinking, your reasons for change,
and all the good stuff out there waiting to help you,
you've everything you need to make it happen.

Just imagine tomorrow being able to say, "I started my
diet yesterday" … that's an achievement!

As I said at the beginning, to help me write this book I needed to go back to Fat-Land ... and I'm still there presently!

Nothing fundamental has changed, and yet some things are quite different.

There are no slim mirrors in Fat-Land, and my size 10 jeans glare at me from the back of the wardrobe.

Fat-land does, however, have loads of elasticated trousers and big pants!

Yet the strangest thing of all is that even though there's unlimited baggage allowance in Fat-Land (you carry your own weight) ... I've nothing to wear because I'm too big!

I look forward to returning to Slim-World, and reading my book completely differently.

A forever kind of diet …

Present day, 2015 …

The journey to Fat-Land was easy. There were no obstacles to overcome. No thinking was required, and it took no time at all. On arrival my life filled up with loads of goodies … endless goodies.

Yes … all of the foods that make me fat were readily available, and could be freely consumed in the name of research!

My buffet table was once again laid out in front of me, only this time there was no calorie counting.

Yippee … bring out the chocolate!

My travel ticket was open ended, and the length of my stay … indeterminate. In my head the big plan was to visit Fat-land for six months.

(As if that was ever going to happen … tee hee!)

In the real world I was to stay for two years!

Where does the time go?

It's hard to believe that the majority of my book was written in 2013, and that two summers, and two Christmas's later, I've been transported to the year 2015!

There was a lot of time to think about *The Thoughtful Diet*.

It had become part of my psyche.

I thought I'd had a purpose, a project, and the end result would see my book finished, completed, finito!

That was my intention … and for a while things were good, I mean really good!

I had given myself a great excuse to overeat. There would be no guilt, and my scales were hidden from view.

All I had to do was enjoy, and learn at the same time.

Things just kept getting better (fatter?), and as time moved on, gradually my size 10 jeans changed into a neat size 16.

Yet still I felt content. The habits of old had returned.

I was so comfy … me and my chocolate, reunited, and so my planned six months became two years!

It was just a matter of time before realisation would hit me, and when it did, it hit me really hard!

I started to feel despair and frustration.

To begin correcting things I knew deep down that all I had to do was follow my own thoughts from the early parts of the book, but still the only image I had of the future was of having to shop for size 18 jeans.

Yikes … something had to happen soon, and it did.

Here's another wee story …

My hubby had booked us a weekend away to Amsterdam, and I had to think about what I needed to take on the trip. By now all my clothes seemed overnight to have shrunk by at least a size. (Maybe that actually happens … tee hee!)

Every time I sat down … no, let's be honest … every time I moved, I seemed to have granted my knickers a kind of superpower. I had somehow given them the ability to transform from being high waist size 16 briefs, to become low rise bikini hipsters. All they had to do was roll down my belly!

Pants that were comfy, and stayed up, were added to the top of my going away list! Big knickers were duly purchased, and me, hubby, and my now size 18's went on our break.

Anyway, Amsterdam came and went and a few weeks later I was helping my mum de-clutter her clothes. My dad always said that every time she opened her wardrobe the theme tune from Dynasty would play.

I opened one of mum's undies drawers, and was mortified to see my pants. The same pants I'd walked the streets of Amsterdam in a few weeks before. How could this be? My clothes were acting weird. I had the same ones at home … had they somehow been transported? Of course not!

Quite simply, I was wearing the same style pants as my 85 year old mother … me … and then came the slap in the face!

Realisation had again hit me hard, and my desire and commitment were back.

My goal was now to search for a way to manage my weight forever, without having to give up the food I love.

This habit of weight off, weight on, would cease to exist.

All I had to do was find my forever kind of diet.

All of us, all of the time, are on a diet. Some of us are on the wrong diet, that's all.

I need to look for the diet that will, at least for now, take me back to Slim-World … so I continue my search.

Meanwhile my mum had continued her dieting programme for two years, even though her daughter had opted out, left her to it, and was eating for Scotland.

Every day she wrote her food diary, and every week she stood on the scales, and at the end of the two years she has lost 3½ lbs in weight.

Ok, on paper that does not seem a lot, but think about it.

I have gained 2½st in the same period by doing absolutely nothing in regard to my weight!

Those of us who seem to be in a constant battle with our weight are always filled with good intentions, and many, many times I intended to "start the diet on Monday"

Choosing that option always gave me the whole weekend to pig out on all the junk food that made me fat in the first place!

How much sense does that make?

Needless to say that by the time my feet hit the floor on Monday morning, I had already decided that maybe it wasn't the best day to actually start … next week would be better … and that choice would give me yet another weekend filled with goodies.

I am so good to myself … not!

Intentions versus chocolate = no contest!

On the subject of good intentions here is a great little quote by John Burroughs …

"The smallest deed is better than the greatest intention"

This wee book of mine may be small in volume, but a lot of time and thought has gone in to it.

It was always my intention to try and remove the waffle, leaving only my thoughts in words that matter.

Happy dieting, and remember …

"Yesterday is history, tomorrow is a mystery, today is a gift, that's why they call it the present".

(Alice Morse Earl, Bill Keane, Winnie the Pooh)

My past lies just ahead of me, and I intend to make sure it's a good one!

At last I can say … I wrote a book, me!

After the book …

June 2015

My forever kind of diet started five weeks ago, and so far I have shed 11½ lbs, and gone down one dress size.

After a lot of thought, and taking everything into account, I chose, coincidentally, Slimming World to help me get back to my Slim-World.

Spooky or what?

Their food optimising diet has caused me to think about the food I eat in a way I have never done before, yet I can still include all my favourites … Eureka!

Mum has lost 4½ lbs in two weeks on the same diet, and at 85 years of age, like me, her thinking in regard to what she's eating has also changed.

My aim is to be vigilant.

The bathroom scales have become my friend, and hand in hand with *The Thoughtful Diet*, they will ensure my life always includes my forever kind of diet.

It seems like ages have passed since I first started writing, and I feel like I've been an 'authoress' forever … ha, ha!

I think when I look back I will have really enjoyed it, but right now I need to sit back and take it all in.

The Thoughtful Diet kept me too busy to do that, so I'm looking forward to tomorrow …

"You are today where your thoughts have brought you. You will be tomorrow, where your thoughts of today take you". *(James Lane Allen)*

Thank you for reading my thoughts!

Good Luck!

Lara Buchanan

Acknowledgements …

Thanks go to my husband, as otherwise the thoughts
would still be in my head.

www.ingramcontent.com/pod-product-compliance
Lightning Source LLC
Chambersburg PA
CBHW040316010626
45792CB00022B/586